COPYRIGHT

Table of contents

Introduction

Do you get cravings, experience persistent lethargy, or do you think you may have a sugar addiction?
Do you occasionally feel unable to face the day when you first awaken?
Most people are trapped on a roller coaster of glucose.
This book will assist you in escaping
The starchy or sugary foods we consume release glucose or blood sugar into our bloodstream.The majority of us have too much glucose in our systems, yet most of us are unaware of this.
This book includes recipes that have been tried and tested by thousands of people who have a question on their minds. It also provides a ground-breaking framework for understanding the function that blood sugar and glucose surge play in general health.

MORE ENERGY.LESS CRAVINGS.LES MID-DAY SNACKING .BETTER SKIN.POSITIVE CHANGE AND HORMONAL BALANCE.A BETTER NIGHT'S SLEEP THAN EVER.

Because the approach makes sense and yields result within shortest time and people are able to maintain the recipes and other healthy living practices outlined in this book.The best part is that you won't have to worry about managing calories and can have all of your favorite meals, like the ideal fish for breakfast or no-spike fiber.
Start your meal with a vegetable, such as broccoli.

One of the most effective methods to enhance your health is to balance your blood sugar, and the glucose Aid is here to make it simple, enjoyable, sweet, and easy.

Chapter 1

What is glucose?

Glucose is the most common form of sugar in the blood and the primary source of energy for the body's cells.

There are many different types and forms of caloric sweeteners that are collectively called "sugar." The most familiar type of sugar is table sugar.

Scientifically speaking, table sugar is sucrose, a disaccharide made of equal parts of two monosaccharides:
"fructose and glucose".

Monosaccharides are single units of sugar and are often referred to as "simple" sugars. The three main monosaccharides that we consume are fructose, galactose and glucose.

They combine in various pairs to form the three kinds of disaccharides (two linked sugar units) that are most important in human nutrition: lactose, maltose and sucrose.

Glucose is the common thread in each of these. It is part of sucrose (linked with fructose), lactose (linked with galactose),

and maltose, which consists of two linked glucose units.

In addition to glucose being integral to disaccharides,

It is also necessary for life.

 Our body uses glucose primarily for energy, and some tissues, including the brain, need a steady supply of glucose as well .
 Since glucose flows in our bloodstream as a readily available energy source, it is referred to as "blood sugar."
The body stores it as glycogen to be used as a source of energy when the blood supply of glucose may be insufficient.

Chapter 2

What is the source of glucose?

The glucose isthe most prevalent
monosaccharide in the world.
It is produced by photosynthesis in plants.

Chains of glucose are stored by some plants and
it is called Starch.

Some of the foods that contains starch include :
- corn
- potatoes
- rice
- wheat.

From these entire food sources, starch is
professionally separated to create dextrose,

glucose, maltodextrins, polyols, and high fructose corn syrup, which are then used as ingredients in the creation of a variety of foods, drinks and sauces.

Honey and dried fruits including dates, apricots, raisins, currants, cranberries, prunes, and figs are the two sources of glucose monosaccharides that are found in the highest concentration in whole foods.

Chapter 3

Is glucose added or natural sugar?

Depending on where it comes from, the sugar we eat is either referred to as natural sugar or added sugar.

If glucose is taken straight from whole foods like apricots and dates, it is regarded as a natural sugar.

When consumed from packaged foods and beverages to which it has been added during manufacture, glucose is regarded as an added sugar. Sadly, just approximately one in ten persons in America consumes the recommended daily amounts of fruits and vegetables, while six out of ten consume more added sugars than is healthy.

Can the body produce glucose?

Glucose is necessary for our bodies to function.

Given that our brain consumes roughly 60% of the glucose than our bodies consume, it is very important for this organ.
 But glucose doesn't always have to come from food and drink right away.

The body produces its own glucose to make sure we always have plenty.

By dissolving glycogen to release the glucose it contains, this can be accomplished. Between meals or during times of vigorous exercise, glycogen is broken down.

The process of gluconeogenesis, which is mostly carried out by the liver, allows the body to create glucose from non-carbohydrate sources.

When glycogen reserves are depleted and glucose ingestion is inadequate or nonexistent, gluconeogenesis takes place, for instance, when in famine or extended fasting.

Chapter 4

Metabolism of Glucose

When we ingest carbs, they break down into simple sugars, which all combine to form glucose, which then travels through the blood to the cells.

A signal for the pancreas to create insulin is sent once the concentration of glucose increases around the cells.
once within the cell, the insulin finds its way to the insulin receptors.
The message is then translated and transmitted to the DNA by the nuclear receptors (PPARs) after being received by the signal in the cell.

The cell membrane is then approached by glucose protein transporters, which pierce it to allow glucose to enter the cell.

Chapter 5

The Role of cell In Glucose Metabolism

When your cells eat, glucose—a compound made of fructose and galactose—is the main source of fuel.

Although the mechanism by which your cells consume glucose is not difficult, there are a few general facts about cells that you need be aware of in order to properly comprehend this process.

The first thing to understand is that a membrane comprised of fat surrounds each and every one of our cells. The necessary fatty acids omega 6 and 3 make up the type of fat found incell membranes. The strength of the cell is guaranteed by this fatty acid.

The membrane will flex but won't break even though it is malleable and impermeable.

These membrane contains insulin receptors, which are receptor sites.Vitamin E, magnesium, chromium, and vanadium are just a few of the vitamins and minerals that make up these receptors.

This is where the insulin lands to provide its signal to the cell, as suggested by the name.

Every cell contains a nucleus.
Other receptors known as PPAR receptors can be found in the nucleus,because they receive the insulin signal and convert it into DNA language, these receptors are more like translators.
 One of the hormones made in the pancreas is insulin.

What occurs when the body is unable to metabolize glucose

The strength of the cell will be harmed and it will die if the cell membrane dries out and loses its fatty acids.

This can be inherited or the effect of unsound eating practices.
Some of the vitamins and minerals that make up the insulin receptors may be lacking.

They won't be able to communicate clearly as a result.
This can be a result of starvation or a genetic tendency.
this process could lead to any of the above-mentioned symptoms as a result of faulty glucose metabolism.

The three can be addressed with food and vitamins if discovered in time.
If the cell membrane dries out and loses its fatty acids, the integrity of the cell will be compromised, and the cell will eventually die.

This could be genetic or the result of unhealthy eating habits.

The insulin receptors may be deficient in some of the vitamins and minerals that make them up. As a result, they won't be able to speak clearly.

Starvation or a hereditary predisposition may be to blame for this.
The PPARs are made of linoleic acid, an omega-6 fatty acid.

Blood sugar levels might be balanced or can spike depending on our dietary choices and lifestyle habits.
Pre-diabetes and type 2 diabetes are both increasing quickly in North America,

Chapter 6

How Do glucose Levels Change?

The body converts the carbohydrates we
consume into glucose, or sugar.

The bloodstream then absorbs this sugar, which is
used to produce energy.
The pancreas releases the hormone insulin,
which controls this process.
Your liver stores any extra blood sugar that is not
needed by the body for energy.

Everything is carefully planned so you have
energy when you need it.
if your insulin levels are balanced appropriately, of
course! What if they aren't, though? Diabetes and
blood sugar dysregulation appear at that point.

Chapter 7

Indicators of a glucose imbalance

Symptoms of a blood sugar imbalance can include a long list that is frequently simple to attribute to "stress or aging".

These consist of:
- Extra abdominal fat:
  Your body releases more insulin when it detects high glucose levels in an effort to get your cells to start absorbing the extra glucose.

  Insulin promotes fat storage, especially around the abdomen. Unfortunately, since belly fat promotes insulin resistance, your pancreas subsequently reacts by releasing even more insulin, which can lead to a vicious cycle.

Do you frequently "crash" after a meal high in carbohydrates? Or when you don't eat for a time, do you get queasy, cranky, or "hungry"? Mood swings, including spurts of frenzied energy followed by sharp drops in energy, are frequently caused by blood sugar changes and a diet that spikes blood sugar quickly.

- desires: Another annoying irony is that desires for more carb- and sugar-rich meals increase when blood sugar levels are too high, which feeds the cycle of insulin production.

  This indicates that there may be a gastrointestinal problem in addition to the uneven blood sugar levels.

- Inability to concentrate: Without the glucose-derived energy, brain cells don't work as well.

  Concentration and focus suffer as a result, yet eating anything that spikes your blood sugar levels isn't the answer because you'll collapse later.

- Thyroid issues: There is a complicated relationship between insulin and thyroid health.

  The thyroid might suffer from too much insulin. A healthy thyroid also aids in the regulation of insulin.

- Unhealthy female hormones are dependent on stable blood sugar levels.

In other words, when insulin levels are too high, more testosterone is produced, and the tissue in the belly fat tissue turns extra testosterone into estrogen.
 As a result, the body makes more estrogen than it needs, which lowers progesterone levels, because progesterone is a relaxing hormone, women who have low levels of it frequently experience symptoms of:
sadness
sleeplessness, Anxiety, and other condition.

Chapter 8

Diseases attributed to excessive glucose

A chronic rise in blood glucose levels is caused by a lack of glucose homeostasis.

Chronic superphysiological glucose concentration, in contrast to physiological glucose concentration which has a deleterious impact on a variety of organs and tissues caused by persistent hyperglycemia

Glucose toxicity refers to a decrease in insulin secretion and an increase in insulin resistance.

It is now widely acknowledged that glucose toxicity influences cell secretion, which contributes to the progression of diabetes.

The harmful effects of hyperglycemia have been explained by a number of different mechanisms.

It was discovered that a persistent hyperglycemia causes neutrophils' declining function.

Thus, the primary issue brought on by acute glucose poisoning is infection. In other words, ongoing hyperglycemia poses a risk for fatal outcomes in both chronic and acute conditions.

it becomes a risk factor for infection, especially during the perioperative period and during the acute phase.Chronic hyperglycemia is a sign of diabetes, and the primary cause of diabetic complications, which may appear several years after the onset of the illness

Since hyperglycemia itself decreases the ability of pancreatic B-cells to secrete insulin and the ensuing rise in insulin resistance results in continued hyperglycemia, glucose toxicity, in its restricted definition, can imply a clinical situation where control of diabetes in particular is inadequate.

Finally, this vicious cycle renders B-cells completely unable to release insulin.

On the other hand, numerous organs are known to be damaged by acute hyperglycemia, which is similar to chronic hyperglycemia.

The acute phase of hyperglycemia impairs neutrophil function and increases the risk of infection throughout the perioperative period. We will introduce the numerous processes known to be involved in the regulation of glucose homeostasis and the emergence of glucose toxicity in this book.

The brain and muscles consume glucose more often than other tissues, metabolic fuels are kept in reserve for usage when needed to ensure that the brain and other tissues always have access to glucose. In addition several insulin-like growth factors, the anabolic hormone insulin plays a major role in regulating glucose homeostasis

The term "anti-insulin"

 Anti insulin or "counter-regulatory hormones" refers to a group of catabolic hormones that may counteract the effects of insulin, including catecholamines, cortisol, growth hormone, and adrenocorticotropic hormone.

Even when diabetes is not a factor, it is frequently discovered that critically sick individuals develop hyperglycemia due to insulin resistance.

The neuroendocrine system responds to stress by increasing the release of anti-insulin hormones, which causes insulin resistance and a decrease in insulin secretion.

As a result, the liver's glucogenesis, adipose tissue's lipolysis, and skeletal muscle's protein catabolism are all increased. Surgical diabetes is the term for this.

Diabetes patients are more vulnerable to stress and are more likely to experience an exacerbation of their condition,which raises the likelihood ofcomplications.

Chapter 9

THE GLUCOSE TOXICITY MECHANISM

It has been discovered that the fundamental cause of glucose toxicity, decreased insulin production and secretion, is related to oxidative stress at the molecular level.

The pancreas may be more vulnerable to oxidative stress than other tissues and organs because pancreatic islet cells exhibit exceptionally limited antioxidative enzyme manifestation.

oxidative stress production pathway
Reactive oxygen species (ROS), such as superoxides (O_2-), hydroxyl radicals ($OH-$), peroxyl radicals ($ROO-$), and nitric oxide, are continuously produced by metabolic processes.

ROS play a role in a variety of biological processes, including atherosclerosis, inflammation, carcinogenesis, and aging.

However, a number of antioxidant enzymes support the maintenance of low ROS levels. The overproduction of ROS, which can harm cellular components including lipids, proteins, or DNA is referred to as oxidative stress. Strong evidence suggests that oxidative stress play a major role in diabetic complications

The oxidative stress markers heme oxygenase-1, 4-hydroxy-2-nonenal, and 8-hydroxy-2-deoxyguanosine (8-OHdG), which are all elevated in the pancreatic islet cells of type 2 diabetes mellitus animal models during laboratory investigation research are also reported to be elevated in patients with type 2 diabetes mellitus Diabetes-related ROS production appears to be directly correlated with long-term hyperglycemia.

It is believed that a number of processes contribute to the rise in oxidative stress in a hyperglycemic state
because a non-enzymatic glycosylation reaction (glycation) is amplified in the hyperglycemic state, the first pathway experiences increase oxidative stress as a result of hyperglycemia.

The intermediate metabolite Amadori compound subsequently produces ROS, which in turn triggers a glycation reaction that produces metabolites known as advanced glycosylation end products.

The mitochondrial electron transport system is another mechanism that can lead to oxidative stress.

This mechanism is found in the inner membrane of the mitochondria, which is where adenosine triphosphate, a significant organic energy source, is made.

Water molecules are produced in this electron transfer mechanism by the deoxidation of four of the oxygen molecules'
 ROS is created as a byproduct of this action, and part of the ROS escape from the system.

Even in normal settings, a portion of the oxygen required for this activity is created as superoxide anions, and their production rises in the hyperglycemic state.

Also contributing to oxidative stress is the hexosamine pathway.
It was discovered that oxidative stress is also caused by glucosamine, an intermediate metabolite in this process.

In fact, it is well recognized that chronically elevated glucose concentrations can cause oxidative stress in primary adipocyte cells and it was shown that oxidative stress prevents Glut 4 from moving to the plasma membrane, which results in insulin resistance in the 3T3-L1 adipocyte cell line

Diabettes Complicates at Glucose Toxicity
  Due to :
- Age
- obesity
- Sedentary lifestyles
- population expansion.

Diabetes mellitus prevalence is alarmingly rising globally. As a result, diabetes problems are also rising.

The most crucial aspects of general diabetes patient care are seen to be complication prevention and treatment.

Complications are primarily brought about by chronic hyperglycemia, which damages numerous organs and creates abnormalities in tissue metabolism.

The top diabetes side effects are mentioned in below.
Depending on the progression of the condition, they are classified as "chronic or acute consequences"

persistent tissues, Vascular tissue suffers the most damage when metabolic abnormalities brought on by diabetes are left untreated for a long time.

Chronic complications are separated into macrovascular diseases that are not particular to diabetes but are prevalent and crucial for a prognosis and microvascular diseases that are specific to and common in diabetes.

Numerous fundamental research projects have shown that vasodilative reaction is also hindered in diabetic patients' blood vessels, which also affects vascular endothelial cell function.

 Both macrovascular and microvascular diabetes problems might arise because of oxidative stress brought on by hyperglycemia.

Microvascular problems including retinopathy, neuropathy, or nephropathy can be brought on by chronic Hyperglycemia

Since the retina consumes more oxygen and burns more glucose than any other tissue, it is extremely vulnerable to oxidative stres s

Studies on diabetic rat retina and retinal cells exposed to high glucose concentrations have revealed that superoxide concentration is increased.

Oxidative stress has been shown to play a role in both the onset of retinopathy and the persistence of the pathology following normalization of glucose levels in animal models, most likely as a result of persistent ROS.

It is also highly likely that oxidative stress contributes to the emergence of diabetic neuropathy.
Numerous studies have demonstrated the ability of antioxidant enzymes to stop or undo the neurotoxic effects of persistent hyperglycemia.

Additionally, elevated levels of mitochondrial oxidative stress indicators have been found in the urine and kidneys of diabetic rats, suggesting that oxidative stress may play a role in the development of diabetic nephropathy
Additionally, macrovascular consequences from chronic hyperglycemia can occur.

The most common cause of mortality among diabetic people is cardiovascular disease.

it has been unequivocally established that chronic hyperglycemia in diabetic and pre-diabetic states is associated with a higher risk of cardiovascular disease development

The risk of cardiovascular, cerebrovascular, and peripheral arterial disorders was reported to be significantly increased by the long-term incubation of macrovessels with high concentrations of glucose.

Since it causes: alteration of contractile protein protein kinase C activation by hyperglycemia is thought to have a major role in vascular problems

Nitric oxide synthase activity rising, nitric oxide synthase Angiotensin-converting enzyme (ACE) activation.

Cardiomyocytes and endothelial cells have been shown to undergo apoptosis and necrosis when ACE is activated

Studies suggesting that inhibiting ACE can protect against cardiovascular diseases.
have confirmed the significance of ACE in the development of cardiovascular disease.

Finally, protein glycation is another element that cardiovascular disorders may emerge from.

Numerous perioperative issues such as

Cardiac problems

neurological infectious complications, might be made worse by hyperglycemia.
Treatment for hyperglycemia generally leads to better outcomes

There are type of consciousness disruption known as a diabetic coma and it's typical of diabetes in its acute state.

These three types of diabetic coma exist:

- Lactic acidosis, Non-ketotic
- Hyperosmolar coma
- ketoacidotic coma brought on by hyperglycemia.

A clinical condition known as infection in acute complications is not unique to diabetic conditions, although it can readily worsen them.

Due to their impaired immune systems and increased bactericidal activity, diabetes individuals need extra care because their infection foci spread considerably more quickly than those of non-diabetic patients.

Particularly in the domains of surgery, emergency, and critical care medicine, this becomes a concern.

Infection and hyperglycemia are related
The promotion of wound healing by perioperative adequate glucose management has been proven.

Infections at the surgical site and other perioperative infectious problems are significant postoperative consequences.

In comparison to individuals with normal HbA1c levels, those with preoperatively elevated HbA1c levels have been shown to have a considerably greater risk of surgical site infections.

Recent fundamental studies have discovered that a hyperglycemic state is what causes the functional loss of neutrophils, indicating that decreased chemotaxis, phagocytic activity, and bactericidal capacity are contributing factors as well as increased adhesive capacity.

Blood glucose levels rise proportionately to a reduction in neutrophil function, with 200 mg/dL being thought to be the cutoff point for neutrophil dysfunction.

In a patient group whose blood glucose level was maintained below 200 mg/dL by insulin injection, the incidence of deep sternal wound infection dropped from 2.0% to 0.8%, according to Furnary et al, With other instances of lower infectious risk due to stringent glycemic control Since the stress response is a risk factor for postoperative infection, maintaining a perioperative hyperglycemic state is crucial for postoperative infection prevention.

importance of maintaining blood glucose levels

Blood sugar balance is essential because it can impact your energy levels, weight gain or loss, mental function, and mood, blood sugar balance is crucial.

The pancreas produces the hormones called insulin, which control blood sugar [or glucose] levels.

The sugars and carbohydrates in food and beverages cause a natural rise in blood sugar when you eat or drink them.

After that, your insulin will start working hard to keep your blood sugar levels stable, your body will release too much insulin if you eat too much sugar or too many carbohydrates [that will turn into sugar] too rapidly.

This is due to the fact that your blood sugar levels are rising too quickly at the time and just in case you weren't aware:Hyperglycemia is what you experience when your blood sugar levels are excessively high.

You may experience what's referred to as hypoglycemia when they're too low.
An imbalanced diet and particular lifestyle patterns lead to blood sugar abnormalities in many otherwise healthy persons:

- Your energy levels
- sleep

- moods
- physical performance will all be improved by maintaining a lifestyle that prevents blood sugar abnormalities.

Additionally, it can stop the onset of insulin resistance and a number of related chronic illnesses.

Signs of glucose Imbalance

To maintain optimal physical function, your brain must receive the proper amount of glucose.

Maintaining a stable blood sugar range is crucial because if your levels are too high or too low, your brain may stop working properly.

The range of "normal" blood sugar is between 70 and 140 mg/dl.
When blood sugar falls below 55 mg/dL, a person experiences clinical hypoglycemia, which causes symptoms like:

- Fatigue
- Dizziness
- Difficulty focusing, Disorientation
- Blurred vision
- Hunger
- Shakiness
- An accelerated heart rate, Anxiety
- Perspiration.

The situation might be complicated; some people may have low blood sugar yet not have any symptoms.

This can also be impacted by things like eating too much or too little sweets.
These are only a few signs that your sugar intake is either excessive or insufficient.

 Both can be brought on by an imbalanced diet for many people who have blood sugar abnormalities.
until you balance your diet, this can result in symptom swings that may appear inexplicable.

Do you want to know why some signs of blood sugar abnormalities happen?

Here is some further information regarding some of the most typical signs of ongoing blood sugar imbalances:

Depression, anxiety, and moodiness

- Do you frequently experience anxiety or depression?

- Is your temperament suddenly fluctuating but you don't know why?

Because glucose is your brain's main source of fuel (or that of excess sugars), it stands to reason that it might react adversely if you don't provide it with enough of it.

It has been demonstrated that glycemic control and mental health symptoms are related.

Anxiety, anger, and depression are all signs of glucose regulation problems.
You can discover that such symptoms disappear by controlling the glucose levels in your body.

Some of these symptoms may be relieved with dietary and lifestyle modifications.

However, it's a good idea to speak with a healthcare provider if you're having trouble managing your mental health,having trouble losing weight or observing extra belly fat

Pre-diabetes and type 2 diabetes have major side effects that can affect the

- Heart
- Nerves
- Kidneys
- Eyes

- Kidney disease.

Understand and manage your blood sugar levels right away because your body will thank you for it.

Experience Cravings for Sugar
You should know by now that one of your body's main fuel sources is blood sugar, also known as glucose.

It is essential to your body's daily operations. Sugar cravings are frequently caused by low blood sugar since your body isn't receiving enough energy to perform correctly,your brain will overcompensate as a result and inform you that you require more sugar than you actually do.

After eating carbs do you feel tired?

Foods high in carbohydrates can frequently cause a groggy feeling after eating.
When carbohydrates are broken down into sugar, a substance called serotonin is released.

Your brain releases serotonin, which is a crucial neurotransmitter for happiness.
Uncontrollable Hunger Your brain is immediately impacted by low blood sugar levels and as a result.

Cortisol or adrenaline may be released by your brain. To boost your blood sugar levels and rebalance your body, your brain performs this.
 So the chemical response that gives rise to the feeling of hunger is brought on by low blood sugar levels in your body.

Your body's ability to Balance Blood Sugar is Affected by a Number of Factors

Chapter 10

Ellements that will affect your body's capacity to correctly manage glucose levels include the following:

- Having a weight issue:
  If you have too much visceral fat, your body may not produce enough insulin to function correctly.

  Insulin resistance may develop as a result over time.

- A diet that is out of balance:
  having an excessively high or excessively low calorie diet
  An unbalanced diet can cause protracted periods of blood sugar imbalance because it

contains either too many or too little carbohydrates and sugars.

- Stress:
  Especially prolonged stress may result in the production of hormones that raise your blood sugar levels.

- Vitamin deficiencies have been linked to diabetes. Think about Vitamin D, magnesium, and chromium.
  You may want to think about taking supplements if your diet does not provide you with the appropriate amount of vitamins.
  before including any supplements in your diet, don't forget to talk to your doctor.

- Having a sedentary lifestyle: Blood sugar levels can be lowered by exercise for up to 24 hours thereafter.
  If you don't have a regular workout schedule and your blood sugar is too high.

- Inconsistent sleep patterns: Your body uses the time you spend sleeping to adjust your hormone levels.
  If you don't get enough sleep, your brain might tell you to eat more sugar to make up for your lack of energy.

- Testing for Imbalances:
  The following are some of the most used methods for testing and monitoring blood sugar levels.

- Blood Sugar Monitor:

When considering checking your blood sugar levels, blood glucose meters frequently spring to mind first.

You must pick up a finger and apply a blood sample to a test strip in order to use this device.
Monitoring of Continuous glucose, the most precise and thorough technique to start comprehending any blood glucose level is likely to be using continuous glucose monitoring (CGMs).

CGMs are put to your skin and left there for roughly two weeks while they continuously monitor your blood sugar levels.

 The Nutrisense CGM allows you to track and monitor your blood sugar swings throughout the day by displaying those data points in a cutting-edge app.

- Test of urine:
Blood sugar levels can also be accurately measured via urine testing. You must dip a test strip into a sample of urine.

Though it is one of the least accurate ways to check your blood sugar levels due to the requirement for a new urine sample, it may also be one of the most uncomfortable.

- AIC Test

AIC testing is a procedure carried out in a lab.

A blood sample will be taken by your doctor, and the lab will review the results for you.

Chapter 11

The 18 Best Foods for glucose Control

- Broccoli Fish
- Seafood
- A pumpkin nut
- Nuts
- Okra
- Flaxseed
- Lentil with beans
- Chia nut
- Kale
- Berries
- Avocado
- Oat and oat grain
- Citrus

- Yoghurt and kefir

- magnesium and chromium content food.

- Apples

- Fibre

- Water

1.Broccoli Fish:

Sources of glucosinolates concentrated in broccoli sproutsinclude glucoraphanin.

According to research, taking these substances as a supplement in the form of a powder or extract can assist persons with type 2 diabetes improve their insulin sensitivity and lower their blood sugar levels.

Consuming cruciferous vegetables may also lower your chance of developing type 2 diabetes, although more research is required

Eat broccoli and sprouts raw or lightly steamed, or prepare them with active sources of myrosinase, such as mustard seed powder.

2. Seafood:

A valuable source of protein, good fats, vitamins, minerals, and antioxidants that may help control blood sugar levels is seafood, which includes fish and shellfish.

Protein is crucial for controlling blood sugar.It promotes sluggish digestion, reduces blood sugar surges after meals, and heightens feelings of satiety. Also it could aid in preventing overeating and encourage the elimination of extra body fat, both of which are necessary for maintaining appropriate blood sugar levels.

It has been demonstrated that consuming a lot of fatty fish, such salmon and sardines, can aid with blood sugar management.

In a small trial with 68 participants, for instance, persons with overweight or obesity who had 26 ounces (oz), or 750 grams (g), of fatty fish each week experienced significant reductions in postmeal blood sugar levels in comparison to those who ingested lean fish.

3. pumpkin seeds and pumpkin:The vibrantly colored, fiber- and antioxidant-rich pumpkin is a fantastic option for controlling blood sugar levels.

Many nations use pumpkin as a traditional treatment for diabetes.Polysaccharides, a type of carb, are abundant in pumpkin.They have been investigated for their potential to control blood sugar.

In small-scale human investigations as well as experiments on animals, treatments using pumpkin extracts and powders have been proven to considerably lower blood sugar levels.

Pumpkin seeds are a great option for blood sugar a control group since they are full of protein and good fats

4.Nut butter and nuts: Nut consumption has been linked to potential benefits for controlling blood sugar levels, according to research.

5. Okra :A fruit that is frequently utilized as a vegetable is okra. It has a lot of substances that reduce blood sugar, like polysaccharides and flavonoid antioxidants.

Okra seeds have powerful blood sugar-lowering properties, making them useful as a natural diabetic treatment.

The primary polysaccharide in okra, rhamnogalacturonan, has been discovered to possess potent anti-diabetic properties. Additionally, the flavonoids isoquercitrin and quercetin 3-O-gentiobioside found in okra can lower blood sugar by inhibiting some enzymes

6. Flaxseed: Flaxseed has a high content of good fats and fiber, which may help lower blood sugar levels.

In an 8-week study of 57 persons with type 2 diabetes, those who had plain yogurt instead of 7 oz (200 g) of 2.5% fat yogurt with 1 oz (30 g) of flaxseed daily saw substantial increases in HbA1c, a marker of long-term blood sugar management.

7. Lentils with beans: Magnesium, fiber, and protein are all abundant in beans and lentils. These vitamins and minerals reduces blood sugar.

 They are especially rich in soluble fiber and resistant starch, which aid in slowing digestion and may enhance the response of blood sugar to meals.

For instance, a research involving 12 women found that adding black beans or chickpeas to a rice meal dramatically lowered blood sugar levels after eating 8. Korean and sauerkraut food

Probiotics, antioxidants, and minerals are among the ingredients found in fermented foods like kimchi and sauerkraut. These substances have been linked in studies to increased insulin sensitivity and blood sugar control .

8. Chia nut :Consuming chia seeds helps to regulate blood sugar. Consuming chia seeds lowers blood sugar levels and increase insulin sensitivity, according to some research.

9 . Kale: Kale is frequently referred to as a "superfood" and for good reason.

It contains a variety of substances, such as fiber and flavonoid antioxidants, that may lower blood sugar levels.

According to a study involving 42 Japanese people, eating either 7 or 14 grams of kale with a high-carb dinner significantly reduced post-meal blood sugar levels compared to a placebo.

 Quercetin and kaempferol, two flavonoid antioxidants present in kale, have been demonstrated in studies to have significant impacts on decreasing blood sugar and insulin sensitivity.

10. Berries :   vNumerous studies relate eating berries to better blood sugar control.

Berries are a great option for people who have trouble controlling their blood sugar because they are high in fiber, vitamins, minerals, and antioxidants.

In comparison to a control group, persons with prediabetes who consumed 2 cups (250 g) of red raspberries with a high-carb meal experienced significantly lower postmeal insulin and blood sugar levels.

Studies have revealed that strawberries, blueberries, and blackberries—in addition to raspberries—benefit blood sugar control by boosting insulin sensitivity and enhancing glucose clearance from the blood

 11. Avocados :Avocados may have important advantages for controlling blood sugar.

They are a good source of fiber, vitamins, minerals, and healthy fats, and include them in meals may help with blood sugar regulation.

12. Oats and oat grain: Due to their high solvent fiber content, which has been shown to have significant glucose lowering capabilities, oats and oat grain should be included in your diet in order to help you manage your glucose levels.

13. Citrus: Citrus organic products are classified as having a low to medium glycemic index even though they do include conventional sugar. Also excellent sources of fiber, minerals, and nutrients are citrus natural goods.

Organic citrus fruit contains plant compounds such naringenin, a polyphenol with potent

anti-diabetic activities, and is high in fiber.
Oranges and grapefruit are two examples of citrus
fruit.

14.yogurt and kefir: Fermented dairy products
like kefir and yogurt may be able to control blood
sugar levels.

Kefir is a probiotic-rich yogurt drink that has been
shown in an 8-week study of 60 patients with type
2 diabetes to dramatically lower fasting blood
sugar and HbA1c when compared to kefir that
does not include probiotics.

Consuming yogurt reduces the risk of type 2 diabetes as well.

Protein, good fats, vitamins, minerals, and antioxidants are all abundant in eggs. Consuming eggs has been associated with better blood sugar control in some studies.

15.Ingest foods high in magnesium and chromium.

Micronutrient deficiencies have been linked to diabetes and high blood sugar levels. Deficits in the minerals magnesium and chromium are a few examples.

The metabolism of carbohydrates and fats involves chromium. It might enhance the effects of insulin, which would help with blood sugar management.

Foods high in chromium include meats,whole grain items,fruit, veg, and nuts

Blood sugar levels have been demonstrated to be improved by magnesium. In fact, diets high in magnesium are linked to a much lower risk of developing diabetes.

On the other hand, diabetes patients with low magnesium levels may experience insulin resistance and lowered glucose tolerance.

However, if you currently consume a lot of foods high in magnesium and have normal blood magnesium levels, you probably won't benefit from taking a magnesium supplement. Several foods are high in magnesium eg a.Dark-colored leaves

b.pumpkin seeds and squash

c.grains from tuna

d.bananas with dark chocolate

e. avocados

Consuming foods high in chromium and magnesium can lower the risk of deficits and blood sugar issues.

16.Apples: Apples have soluble fiber and plant substances like quercetin, chlorogenic acid, and gallic acid that could help lower blood sugar and prevent diabetes.

Reducing your carb consumption can help with blood sugar regulation. A study of 18 women revealed that eating apples 30 minutes before a rice meal significantly reduced postmeal blood sugar compared to eating rice alone.

17. Consume more fiber: Fiber promotes a more gradual rise in blood sugar by delaying the digestion and absorption of carbohydrates.

Fiber comes in two varieties: soluble and insoluble.Both are crucial, but while insoluble fiber hasn't been specifically demonstrated to help with blood sugar management, soluble fiber has.

A diet rich in fiber can enhance your body's capacity to control blood sugar and reduce blood sugar lows. Among the foods high in fiber are: fruits, vegetables, legumes,whole grains.

For women, a daily fiber intake of 25 grams is advised, while for men it is 35 grams. 14 grams for every 1,000 calories, roughly.

Consuming a lot of fiber can help with blood sugar control. In this regard, soluble dietary fiber seems to be superior to insoluble fiber.

18. Keep hydrated by drinking water:You may be able to maintain healthy blood sugar levels by drinking enough water.

Additionally to avoiding dehydration, it aids in the kidneys' ability to eliminate any extra sugar in the urine.

Drinking water consistently rehydrates the blood, lower blood sugar levels, and lessen the chance of acquiring diabetes, according to one assessment of observational studies, which revealed that people who drank more water had a lower risk of developing high blood sugar levels.

Remember that the greatest beverages are water and others consumeable with no calories. Avoid foods that are sugar-sweetened because they can cause blood sugar to rise, weight gain, and an increased risk of diabetes.

Hydration helps lower blood sugar levels and the risk of developing diabetes.

 Avoid beverages with added sugar and opt instead for water and zero-calorie liquids.

Since it's crucial to stay hydrated so you can eliminate extra glucose through urination, water is always a healthy beverage option for controlling blood sugar. Additionally, your body removes water from other parts of your body when it detects additional glucose, which raises your chance of being dehydrated.

Aim for low-glycemic-index foods.

The glycemic index (GI) gauges:How quickly your body consumes carbohydrates and how quickly they break down after digestion, also how rapidly your blood sugar levels rise is determined by glycemic index (GI).

Foods are classified as low, medium, or high GI according to the GI, which rates them from 0 to 100. The ranking of low GI meals is 55 or lower. .

Foods with a low to moderate GI include, for instance:bulgur barley.Greek yogurt without sugar,Oat,the legumes lentils,vegetables that aren't starchy, whole wheat pasta,Additionally incorporating protein or good fats reduces blood sugar rises

Chapter 12

Other healthy actions that lowers blood glucose level includes:

1. Make an effort to control your stress:Stress can impact the levels of blood sugar in your body. your body releases the hormones glucagon and cortisol in response to stress, which raise blood sugar levels.

Exercise, relaxation, and medication dramatically reduce stress and lowers blood sugar levels, according to a study involving a group of students.

Yoga and mindfulness-based stress reduction are two exercises and relaxation techniques that may help persons with chronic diabetes improve their insulin secretion.

You may be able to control your blood sugar levels by controlling your stress levels through exercise or relaxation techniques like yoga.

2. Get adequate restful sleep:It feels great and is vital for good health to get adequate sleep.

In reality, lack of sleep and poor sleeping patterns can have an impact on insulin sensitivity and blood sugar levels, raising the risk of type 2 diabetes. Additionally, they may boost hunger and encourage weight gain.

Sleep deprivation causes levels of the hormone cortisol to rise, which, as previously mentioned, is crucial for controlling blood sugar.

Getting enough sleep involves both amount and quality. Adults are advised by the National Sleep Foundation to get at least 7-8 hours of good sleep each night.

Try the following to get better sleep:

1.observe a sleeping schedule

2.Stay away from alcohol and caffeine.

3.Lessen your screen time before night.

4.Limit the number of naps you take in your bedroom.

5.Establish a nighttime ritual and utilize relaxing

6.Utilize peaceful and reassuring airfreshners such lavender

7. Avoid working in your bedroom; before bed, take a warm bath or shower; try guided imagery or meditation.

A healthy weight and blood sugar levels are supported by getting enough sleep. On the other side, insufficient sleep might interfere with important metabolic hormones.

8. Think about including particular diet in your food menu.

There are numerous foods and plants that have known therapeutic qualities.

If you already take blood-sugar-lowering drugs, it's imperative to consult your doctor before introducing any of these foods to your diet because some herbal supplements may interact poorly with them.

Finally, unlike how Drug prescription are overseen, the Food and Drug Administration (FDA) does not regulate dietary supplements. As a result, it's critical to buy supplements that have passed an independent lab's tests for ingredient content and purity.

9.Increase your intake of nutritious snacks.

You may be able to avoid having both high and low blood sugar levels by spreading out your meals and snacks throughout the day.

The risk of type 2 diabetes may be decreased by snacking in between meals.

In fact, a number of studies indicate that eating more frequently and in smaller portions throughout the day may increase insulin sensitivity and reduce blood sugar levels.

Snacking in between meals may prevent blood sugar spikes or drops throughout the day.

10. Consume meals high in probiotics

Probiotics are beneficial microorganisms that provide several health advantages, such as better blood sugar management.

According to research, type 2 diabetics who use probiotics may have reduced levels of fasting blood sugar, HbA1c, and insulin resistance.

Interestingly, studies have shown that persons who ingest different species of probiotics and for at least 8 weeks see greater changes in blood sugar levels.

Fermented foods, such as yogurt, are probiotic-rich as long as the label specifies that it contains live active cultures.

tempeh, sauerkraut, and kimchi, a diet high in probiotics aids in controlling blood sugar levels.

11. Various forms of exercise and adequate rest:

Exercise improves insulin sensitivity and makes your muscles more effective at absorbing the glucose they require for energy, both of which contribute to the maintenance of healthy blood sugar levels.

The most effective kind of exercise, according to studies, is high-intensity interval training, but many people find it challenging to maintain that level of intensity on a daily basis.

 Combining physical training with a sort of cardio that you can sustain over time is a great strategy that will maintain hormonal balance and a healthy weight, getting adequate sleep is crucial for blood sugar stabilization.

Unfortunately, having high blood sugar might make it difficult to get a good night's sleep.

Effective Supplements: Herbal supplements can support other blood sugar management therapies,a good example of such supplement is cinnamon, which also has the advantage of providing some sweetness without using sugar

Another simple supplement to include in your diet is ginger, ginseng, probiotics, and aloe vera are some promising supplements: certain foods, such as those that are high in added sugar and refined carbohydrates causes blood sugar oscillations but other foods rich in fibres and vitamin supplements improve blood sugar management while enhancing general health.